The Effortless Comfort Food Guide for Delicious Dishes

The best tasty and affodable comfort food recipe collection

Norman Vega

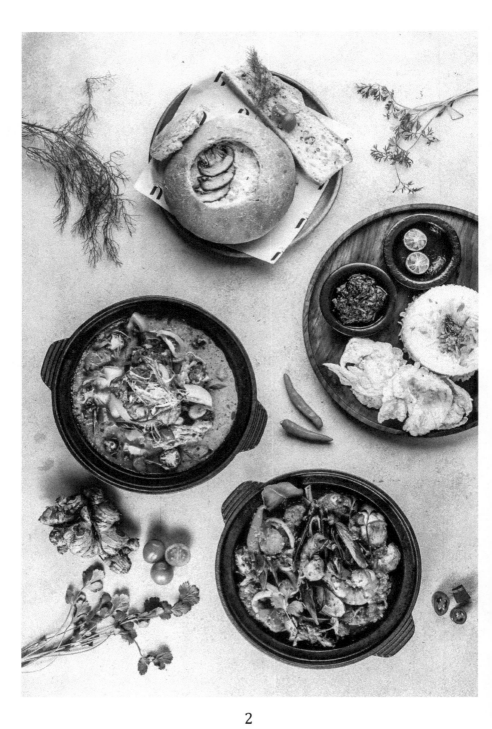

professional advice. The content within this book has been derived from various sources. Please consult a licensed professional before attempting any techniques outlined in this book.

By reading this document, the reader agrees that under no circumstances is the author responsible for any losses, direct or indirect, which are incurred as a result of the use of information contained within this document, including, but not limited to, — errors, omissions, or inaccuracies.

Table of Contents

Meatballs

Preparation Time: 10 minutes | Cooking Time: 20 minutes | Servings: 6

Ingredients:

2 lbs ground beef

1 tsp paprika

1 tsp oregano

1 tsp cinnamon

2 tsp cumin

2 tsp coriander

1 tsp garlic, minced

1 small onion, grated

1 egg, lightly beaten

1 tbsp fresh mint, chopped

1/4 cup fresh parsley, minced

1/2 tsp allspice

1/4 tsp pepper

1/2 tsp salt

Directions:

Add all ingredients into the bowl and mix until combined.

Make small balls from the meat mixture and place them into the Pressure Pot air fryer basket. Place basket in the pot.

Seal the pot air fryer lid and select bake mode and cook at 400° F for 15-20 minutes.

Serve and enjoy.

Nutrition:

Calories 304, Fat 10g, Carbohydrates 2g, Sugar 0.7g, Protein 47g, Cholesterol 162mg.

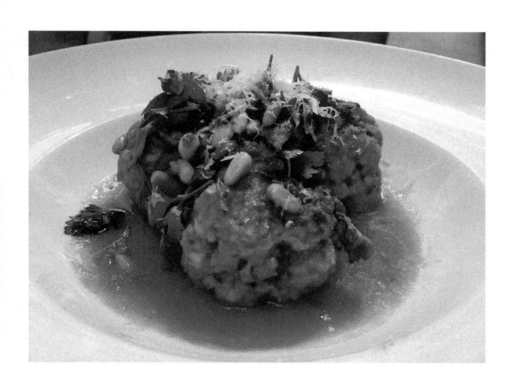

Spicy Lamb Patties

Preparation Time: 10 minutes | Cooking Time: 8 minutes | Servings: 4

Ingredients:

1 lb ground lamb

1/4 cup fresh parsley, chopped

1 tsp dried oregano

1 cup feta cheese, crumbled

1 tbsp garlic, minced

1/4 cup basil leaves, minced

10 mint leaves, minced

1 jalapeno pepper, minced

1/4 tsp pepper

1/2 tsp kosher salt

Directions:

Add all ingredients into the bowl and mix until combined.

Make small patties from the meat mixture and place them into the Pressure Pot air fryer basket. Place basket in the pot.

Seal the pot air fryer lid and select air fry mode and cook at 360° F for 15-18 minutes.

Serve and enjoy.

Nutrition:

Calories 317, Fat 16g, Carbohydrates 3g, Sugar 1.7g, Protein 37g, Cholesterol 135mg.

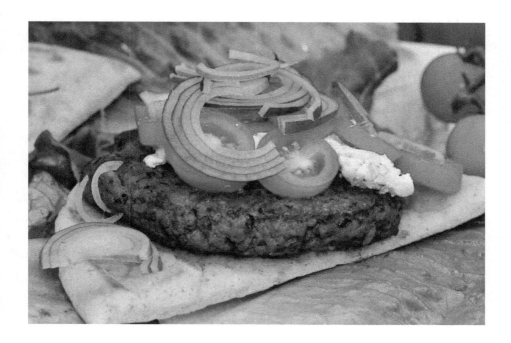

Chuck Roast

Preparation Time: 10 minutes | Cooking Time: 10 hours | Servings: 6

Ingredients:

2 lbs beef chuck roast

2 tbsp balsamic vinegar

1/2 cup beef broth

1/4 cup sun-dried tomatoes, chopped

20 garlic cloves, peeled

1/4 cup olives, sliced

1 tsp Italian seasoning, crushed

Directions:

Place meat into the inner pot of Pressure Pot duo crisp.

Pour remaining ingredients over meat.

Seal the pot with a pressure-cooking lid and select slow cook mode and cook on low for 10 hours.

Remove meat from pot and shred using a fork.

Return shredded meat to the pot and stir well.

Serve and enjoy.

Nutrition:

Calories 578, Fat 43g, Carbohydrates 4g, Sugar 0.5g, Protein 40g, Cholesterol 156 mg.

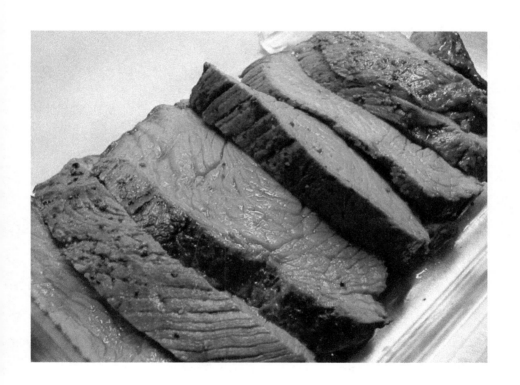

Flavorful Thyme Steak

Preparation Time: 10 minutes | Cooking Time: 10 minutes | Servings: 4

Ingredients:

1 lb flank steak

1/4 cup soy sauce

1 tsp fresh thyme, chopped

1 tbsp lemon zest, grated

2 tbsp olive oil

Pepper

Salt

Directions:

In a mixing bowl, mix soy sauce, thyme, lemon zest, oil, pepper, and salt.

Add steak into the bowl and coat well with soy sauce mixture and let it sit for 10 minutes.

Place the dehydrating tray in a multi-level air fryer basket and place basket in the Pressure Pot.

Place steak on dehydrating tray.

Seal pot with air fryer lid and select air fry mode then set the temperature to 400° F and timer for 10 minutes.

Turn steak halfway through.

Serve and enjoy.

Nutrition:

Calories 290, Fat 16.5g, Carbohydrates 1.7g, Sugar 0.4g, Protein 32.6g, Cholesterol 62mg.

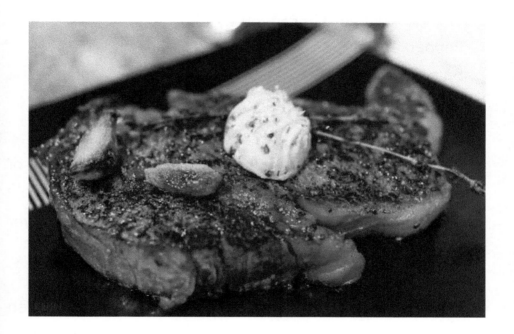

Cheese Stuff Burgers

Preparation Time: 10 minutes | Cooking Time: 8 minutes | Servings: 2

Ingredients:

1 lb ground beef

1 tbsp BBQ seasoning

1/2 cup cheddar cheese, shredded

Pepper

Salt

Directions:

In a bowl, mix meat, BBQ seasoning, pepper, and salt.

Shape patties then stuff some cheese in the center of the patty and wrap the patty around the cheese.

Place the dehydrating tray in a multi-level air fryer basket and place basket in the Pressure Pot.

Place prepared patties on a dehydrating tray.

Seal pot with air fryer lid and select air fry mode then set the temperature to 350° F and timer for 8 minutes.

Turn patties halfway through.

Serve and enjoy.

Nutrition:

Calories 541, Fat 23.6g, Carbohydrates 1.1g, Sugar 0.3g, Protein 76.2g, Cholesterol 233mg.

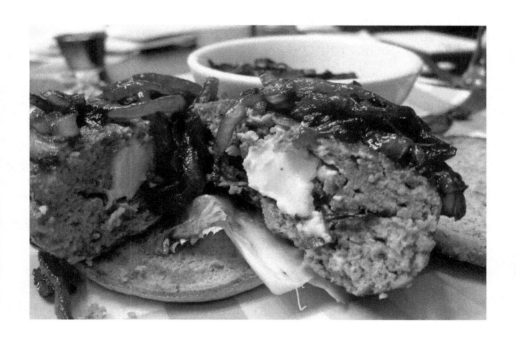

Korean Short Ribs

Preparation Time: 10 minutes | Cooking Time: 10 minutes | Servings: 2

Ingredients:

1 lb beef short ribs

1/4 tsp red pepper flakes

1/2 tbsp ground ginger

1/2 tsp garlic, minced

1/4 cup brown sugar

1/4 cup soy sauce

Directions:

Add ribs with remaining ingredients into the zip-lock bag. Mix well and place in the refrigerator for 1 hour.

Place the dehydrating tray in a multi-level air fryer basket and place basket in the Pressure Pot.

Place marinated ribs on a dehydrating tray.

Seal pot with air fryer lid and select air fry mode then set the temperature to 400° F and timer for 10 minutes. Turn ribs halfway through.

Serve and enjoy.

Nutrition:

Calories 557, Fat 20.6g, Carbohydrates 21.5g, Sugar 18.2g, Protein 67.7g, Cholesterol 206mg.

Asian Meatballs

Preparation Time: 10 minutes | Cooking Time: 12 minutes | Servings: 4

Ingredients:

1 lb ground beef

2 tbsp scallions, chopped

3 tbsp sesame seeds, toasted

1/2 cup Hoisin sauce

1 egg, lightly beaten

1 tsp sugar

2 tsp garlic powder

2 tbsp ginger, grated

1/2 cup breadcrumbs

Directions:

In a mixing bowl, mix meat, egg, sugar, garlic powder, ginger, and breadcrumbs until well combined.

Place the dehydrating tray in a multi-level air fryer basket and place basket in the Pressure Pot.

Make meatballs from meat mixture and place on dehydrating tray.

Seal pot with air fryer lid and select air fry mode then set the temperature to 350° F and timer for 12 minutes. Turn meatballs halfway through.

Transfer meatballs into the large bowl.

Pour hoisin sauce over meatballs and coat well.

Garnish with scallions and sprinkle with sesame seeds.

Serve and enjoy.

Nutrition:

Calories 408, Fat 13.5g, Carbohydrates 29.6g, Sugar 11.2g, Protein 40.4g, Cholesterol 143mg.

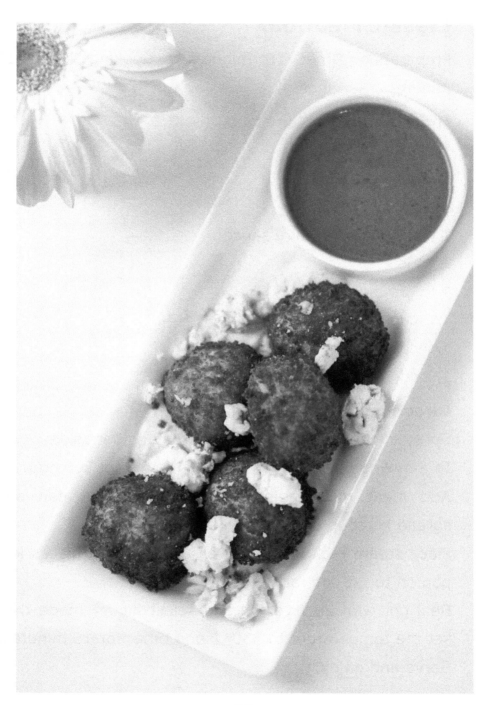

Classic Meatloaf

Preparation Time: 10 minutes | Cooking Time: 15 minutes | Servings: 4

Ingredients:

1 lb ground beef

1 cup breadcrumbs

1 tbsp soy sauce

1 tbsp Worcestershire sauce

2 eggs

1 lb ground pork

1/2 cup green pepper, chopped

1/2 cup onion, chopped

1/3 cup ketchup

Directions:

Spray a loaf pan with cooking spray and set aside.

In a mixing bowl, mix all ingredients except ketchup.

Add meat mixture into the prepared loaf pan and spread ketchup on top.

Place steam rack into the Pressure Pot then places loaf pan on top of the rack.

Seal pot with air fryer lid and select air fry mode then set the temperature to 330° F and timer for 15 minutes. Serve and enjoy.

Nutrition:

Calories 544, Fat 14.8g, Carbohydrates 27.6g, Sugar 8.1g, Protein 71.3g, Cholesterol 266mg.

Easy Meatballs

Preparation Time: 10 minutes | Cooking Time: 10 minutes | Servings: 4

Ingredients:

1 lb ground beef

1/4 cup onion, chopped

1/2 cup breadcrumbs

2 tbsp water

1 egg, lightly beaten

Pepper

Salt

Directions:

Add all ingredients into the large bowl and mix until well combined.

Place the dehydrating tray in a multi-level air fryer basket and place basket in the Pressure Pot.

Make meatballs meat mixture and place on dehydrating tray.

Seal pot with air fryer lid and select air fry mode then set the temperature to 350° F and timer for 10 minutes.

Turn meatballs halfway through.

Serve and enjoy.

Nutrition:

Calories 283, Fat 8.9g, Carbohydrates 10.5g, Sugar 1.2g, Protein 37.7g, Cholesterol 142mg.

Easy Homemade French Fries

Preparation Time: 10 minutes | Cooking Time: 15 minutes | Servings: 4

Ingredients:

2 potatoes, peel & cut into fries' shape

1/2 tsp garlic powder

1/2 tbsp olive oil

Pepper

Salt

Directions:

Soak potato fries in water for 15 minutes. Drain well and pat dry with a paper towel.

Toss potato fries with oil, garlic powder, pepper, and salt.

Add potato fries to an Pressure Pot air fryer basket and place basket in the Pressure Pot.

Seal pot with air fryer lid and select bake mode then set the temperature to 375 ° F and timer for 10 minutes.

Turn fries to the other side and bake for 5 minutes more.

Serve and enjoy.

Nutrition:

Calories 90, Fat 1.9g, Carbohydrates 17g, Sugar 1.3g, Protein 1.9g, Cholesterol 0mg.

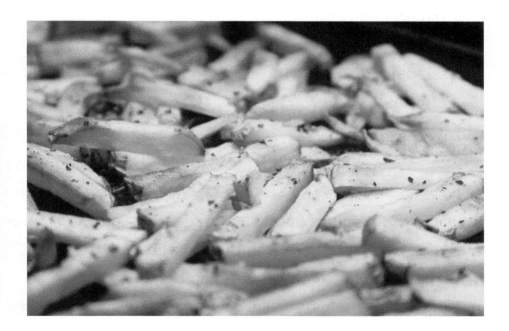

Spicy Cashew Nuts

Preparation Time: 10 minutes | Cooking Time: 5 minutes | Servings: 6

Ingredients:

3 cups cashews

2 tbsp olive oil

1 tsp ground cumin

1 tsp ground coriander

1 tsp paprika

1 tsp salt

Directions:

Add cashews and remaining ingredients into the mixing bowl and toss well.

Place the dehydrating tray in a multi-level air fryer basket and place basket in the Pressure Pot.

Spread cashews on a dehydrating tray.

Seal pot with air fryer lid and select air fry mode then set the temperature to 330° F and timer for 5 minutes.

Serve and enjoy.

Nutrition:

Calories 436, Fat 36.6g, Carbohydrates 22.7g, Sugar 3.5g, Protein 10.6g, Cholesterol 0mg.

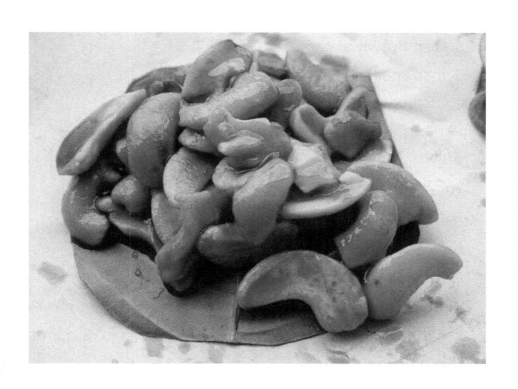

Cinnamon Maple Chickpeas

Preparation Time: 10 minutes | Cooking Time: 12 minutes | Servings: 4

Ingredients:

14 oz can chickpeas, rinsed, drained and pat dry

1 tsp ground cinnamon

1 tbsp brown sugar

1 tbsp maple syrup

1 tbsp olive oil

Pepper

Salt

Directions:

Place the dehydrating tray in a multi-level air fryer basket and place basket in the Pressure Pot.

Spread chickpeas on a dehydrating tray.

Seal pot with air fryer lid and select air fry mode then set the temperature to 375° F and timer for 12 minutes. Stir halfway through.

In a mixing bowl, mix cinnamon, brown sugar, maple syrup, oil, pepper, and salt. Add chickpeas and toss well to coat.

Serve and enjoy.

Nutrition:

Calories 171, Fat 4.7g, Carbohydrates 28.5g, Sugar 5.2g, Protein 4.9g, Cholesterol 0mg.

Parmesan Carrot Fries

Preparation Time: 10 minutes | Cooking Time: 15 minutes | Servings: 4

Ingredients:

4 carrots, peeled and cut into fries

2 tbsp parmesan cheese, grated

1 1/2 tbsp garlic, minced

2 tbsp olive oil

Pepper

Salt

Directions:

Add carrots and remaining ingredients into the mixing bowl and toss well.

Spray Pressure Pot multi-level air fryer basket with cooking spray.

Add carrots fries into the air fryer basket and place basket into the Pressure Pot.

Seal pot with air fryer lid and select air fry mode then set the temperature to 350° F and timer for 15 minutes.

Stir halfway through.

Serve and enjoy.

Nutrition:

Calories 99, Fat 7.6g, Carbohydrates 7.2g, Sugar 3g, Protein 1.6g, Cholesterol 2mg.

Tater Tots

Preparation Time: 10 minutes | Cooking Time: 10 minutes | Servings: 2

Ingredients:

16 oz frozen tater tots

1 tbsp olive oil

Salt

Directions:

Drizzle tater tots with olive oil and season with salt.

Spray Pressure Pot multi-level air fryer basket with cooking spray.

Add tater tots into the air fryer basket and place basket into the Pressure Pot.

Seal pot with air fryer lid and select air fry mode then set the temperature to 400° F and timer for 10 minutes.

Stir halfway through.

Serve and enjoy.

Nutrition:

Calories 492, Fat 28.6g, Carbs 54g, Sugar 1.4g, Protein 5.4g, Cholesterol 0mg.

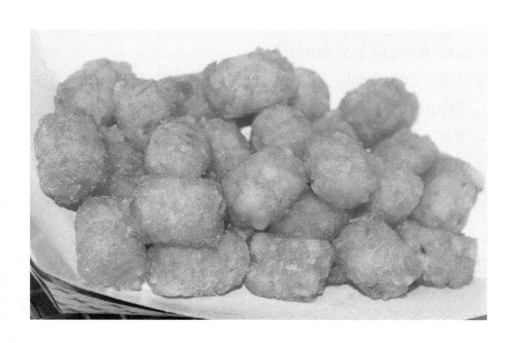

Chili Lime Chickpeas

Preparation Time: 10 minutes | Cooking Time: 12 minutes | Servings: 4

Ingredients:

14 oz can chickpeas, rinsed, drained and pat dry

1 tbsp lime juice

1/4 tsp red pepper

1/2 tsp chili powder

1 tbsp olive oil

Pepper

Salt

Directions:

Add chickpeas, red pepper, chili powder, oil, pepper, and salt into the mixing bowl and toss well.

Place the dehydrating tray in a multi-level air fryer basket and place basket in the Pressure Pot.

Spread chickpeas on a dehydrating tray.

Seal pot with air fryer lid and select air fry mode then set the temperature to 375° F and timer for 12 minutes. Stir halfway through.

Drizzle lemon juice over chickpeas and serve.

Nutrition:

Calories 154, Fat 4.7g, Carbohydrates 24.1g, Sugar 0.6g, Protein 5.1g, Cholesterol 0mg.

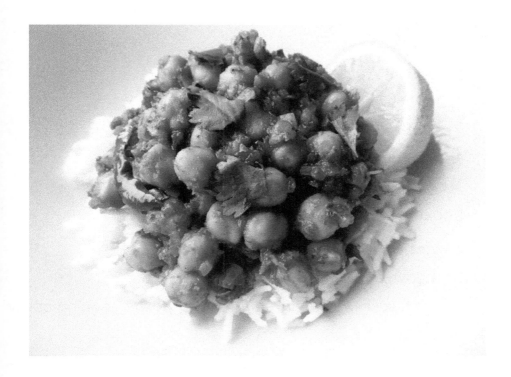

Strawberry Tart

Preparation time: 25 minutes | Cooking Time: 40 minutes | Servings: 8

Ingredients:

1 ½ cups almond flour

1/3 cup butter; melted

2 cups strawberries; sliced

5 egg whites

1/3 cup swerve

Zest of 1 lemon, grated

1 tsp. Baking powder

1 tsp. Vanilla extract

Cooking spray

Directions:

In a bowl, whisk egg whites well.

Add the rest of the ingredients except the cooking spray gradually and whisk everything.

Grease a tart pan with the cooking spray and pour the strawberries mix

Put the pan in the air fryer and cook at 370°f for 20 minutes.

Cool down, slice, and serve

Nutrition:

Calories 182, Fat 12g, Fiber 1g, Carbs 6g, Protein 5g.

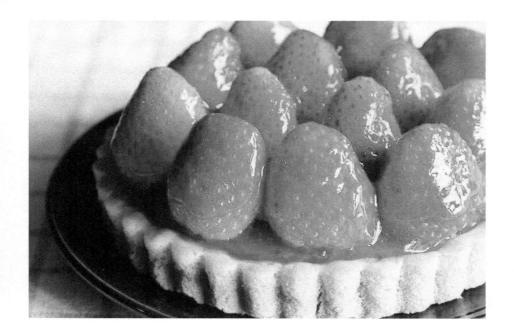

Moroccan-Style Couscous Salad

Preparation time:10 minutes | Cooking Time: 10 minutes

Servings 4

Ingredients:

1-pound couscous

1 tablespoon olive oil

2 tablespoons sesame butter tahini

2 tablespoons fresh mint, roughly chopped

2 bell peppers, diced

1 cucumber, diced

2 cups vegetable broth

1/4 cup yogurt

1 tablespoon honey

2 tomatoes, sliced

A bunch of scallions, sliced

Directions:

Press the "Sauté" button and heat the oil; then, sauté the peppers until tender and aromatic. Stir in the couscous and vegetable broth.

Secure the lid. Choose the "Manual" mode and cook for 2 minutes at high pressure. Once cooking is complete, use a quick pressure release; carefully remove the lid.

Then, stir in the remaining ingredients; stir to combine well and enjoy!

Nutrition:

Calories 563, Fat 9.2g, Carbs 98g, Protein 19.6g, Sugars 7.3g.

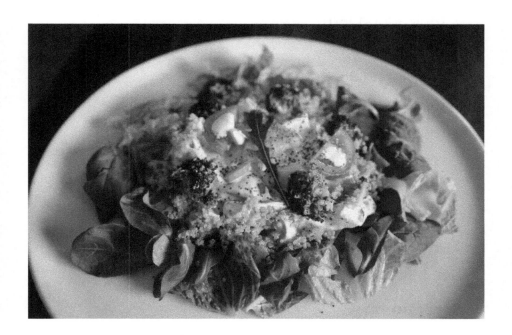

Short Ribs with Herbs and Molasses

Preparation time:1 hour 45 minutes | Cooking Time: 10 minutes

Servings 8

Ingredients:

3 pounds short ribs

1 tablespoon lard

4 cloves of garlic

1 teaspoon cayenne pepper

2 tablespoons rice vinegar

2 tablespoons molasses

2 rosemary sprigs

2 thyme sprigs

1 cup beef bone broth

1/2 cup port wine

Sea salt and ground black pepper, to season

Directions:

Press the "Sauté" button and melt the lard. Once hot, cook the short ribs for 4 to 5 minutes, turning them periodically to ensure even cooking.

Add the other ingredients.

Secure the lid. Choose the "Manual" mode and cook for 90 minutes at high pressure. Once cooking is complete, use a natural pressure release; carefully remove the lid. Afterward, place the short ribs under the broiler until the outside is crisp or about 10 minutes. Transfer the ribs to a platter and serve immediately.

Nutrition:

Calories 372, Fat 27.6g, Carbs 4.9g, Protein 25.7g, Sugars 3.4g.

Popcorn with A Twist

Preparation time:10 minutes | Cooking Time: 10 minutes

Servings 4

Ingredients:

1/2 tablespoon ground cinnamon

1/2 cup popcorn kernels

1/4 cup icing sugar

2 tablespoons coconut oil

Directions:

Press the "Sauté" button and melt the coconut oil. Stir until it begins to simmer.

Stir in the popcorn kernels and cover. When the popping slows down, press the "Cancel" button.

Toss the freshly popped corn with icing sugar and cinnamon. Toss to evenly coat the popcorn and serve immediately.

Nutrition:

Calories 295, Fat 11.5g, Carbs 42.2g, Protein 6.3g, Sugars 6.6g.

Pork Beef Stock Recipe

Preparation Time: 66 minutes | Cooking Time: 10 minutes | Servings: 8

Ingredients:

1-pound beef stew meat

2 lbs. pastured pork bones

1 celery stalk; chopped into thirds

1 small onion; unpeeled and halved

1 tsp. dried bay leaf

1/2 tsp. whole black peppercorns

8 cups of water

1 sprig of fresh parsley

1 tsp. kosher salt

Directions:

Pour the water into the Pressure Pot.

Add all the ingredients to the water.

Secure the lid and turn the pressure release handle to the sealed position.

Select the Manual function; set to high pressure and adjust the timer to 60 minutes,

When it beeps; Natural Release the steam for 10 minutes and remove the lid.

Strain the prepared stock through a mesh strainer and discard all the solids, Skim off all the surface fats and serve hot.

Nutrition:

Calories 464, Carbohydrate 6.7g, Protein 32.1g, Fat 37g, Sugar 0.4g, Sodium 1.57g.

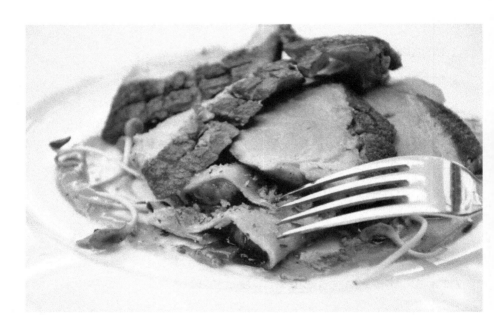

Tomato Basil Sauce Recipe

Preparation Time: 20 minutes | Cooking Time: 10 minutes | Servings: 8

Ingredients:

8 lbs. Romas tomatoes; diced

1 cup chopped fresh basil

4 tbsp. olive oil

1/2 garlic cloves; minced

2 onions; diced

2 tbsp. salt

1 tbsp. pepper

1 tbsp. garlic powder

3 tbsp. Italian seasoning

1/2 tsp. crushed peppers

2 bay leaves

Directions:

Pour the oil into the Pressure Pot and select the **Sauté** function.

Add the garlic and onions to the oil and stir-fry for 5 minutes,

Now add all the remaining ingredients, except the basil to the Pressure Pot.

Secure the lid and turn the pressure release handle to the sealed position.

Select the Manual function; set to high pressure and adjust the timer to 10 minutes,

When it beeps; Quick Release the steam and remove the lid.

Stir well; remove the bay leaves and add the basil to the sauce, Serve.

Nutrition:

Calories 197, Carbohydrate 25.2g, Protein 0.7g, Fat 8.7g, Sugar 15.5g, Sodium 1.43g.

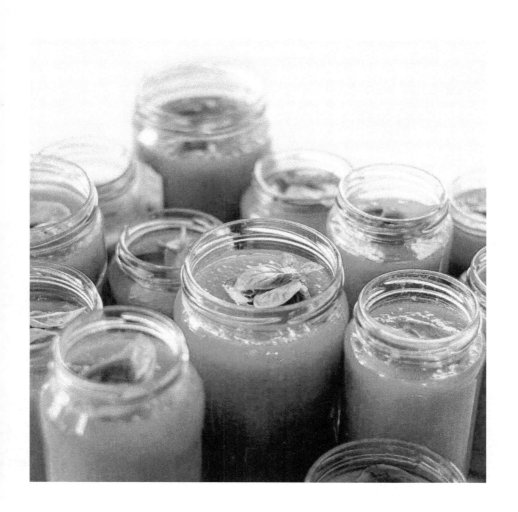

Creamy Hummus

Preparation Time: 10 minutes | Cooking Time: 35 minutes | Servings: 10

Ingredients:

3 cups garbanzo beans, cooked

12 cups water

1/4 tsp paprika

1/2 tsp ground cumin

1 lemon juice

3 garlic cloves

1/4 cup tahini

1/2 cup warm water

1/4 cup olive oil

1 tsp salt

Directions:

Add beans and water into the Pressure Pot.

Seal pot with lid and cook on manual high pressure for 35 minutes.

Once done then allow to release pressure naturally then open the lid.

Drain beans well. Transfer beans into the food processor with remaining Ingredients except for oil and process until smooth.

Add oil and stir well.

Serve and enjoy.

Nutrition:

Calories 300, Fat 12g, Carbohydrates 38.1g, Sugar 6.6g, Protein 12.7g, Cholesterol 0mg.

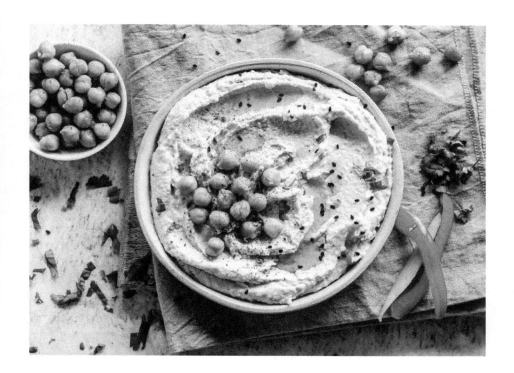

Tomato Pasta Sauce

Preparation Time: 10 minutes | Cooking Time: 45 minutes | Servings: 6

Ingredients:

2 tbsp olive oil

2 tbsp butter

1 lb ground beef

1 small white onion, chopped

5 garlic cloves, minced

6 cups chopped tomatoes

4 tbsp tomato paste

2 cups tomato ketchup

½ cup red wine

½ cup of water

2 bay leaves

2 tsp dried oregano

2 tbsp dried parsley

2 tbsp Italian seasoning

Salt and black pepper to taste

2 tbsp maple syrup

Directions:

Set your Pressure Pot to Sauté mode. Heat olive oil and butter and cook beef until brown, 5 minutes. Add and sauté onion until softened, 3 minutes.

Stir in garlic and cook until fragrant, 30 seconds.

Add tomatoes, tomato paste, tomato ketchup, red wine, water, bay leaves, oregano, parsley, Italian seasoning, salt, black pepper, and maple syrup.

Seal the lid, select Manual/Pressure Cook mode on High, and set the cooking time to 25 minutes. After cooking, perform a natural pressure release for 10 minutes, then a quick pressure release to let out the remaining steam.

Unlock the lid. Stir sauce, turn Pressure Pot off, and allow cooling.

Spoon into jars, cover, and refrigerate.

Use for up to 5 days.

Nutrition:

Kcal 251, Carbs 30g, Fat 13g, Protein 5g.

Mushroom Sauce

Preparation Time: 10 minutes | Cooking Time: 35 minutes | Servings: 6

Ingredients:

5 cups mushrooms, chopped

2 yellow onions, chopped

4 garlic cloves, minced

½ cup chicken broth

1 tsp dried mixed herbs

¼ tsp red chili flakes

1 tsp dried thyme

Salt and black pepper to taste

2 tbsp cornstarch

Directions:

In the inner pot, combine mushrooms, onions, garlic, chicken broth, mixed herbs, chili flakes, thyme, salt, and black pepper. Seal the lid, select Manual/Pressure Cook mode on High, and set the cooking time to 10 minutes. After cooking, perform a natural pressure release for 10 minutes, then a quick pressure release to let out the remaining steam.

Unlock the lid and set it to Sauté mode. Using an immersion blender, puree ingredients until smooth. Stir in cornstarch and allow thickening for 2 to 3 minutes. Spoon soup into bowls and serve.

Nutrition:

Kcal 192; Carbs 15g; Fat 12g; Protein 8g

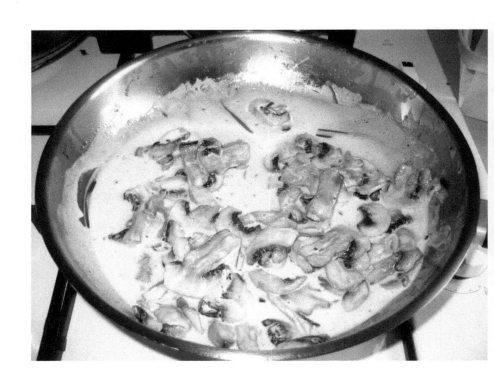

Spinach Dip

Preparation Time: 10 minutes | Cooking Time: 4 minutes | Servings: 10

Ingredients:

1 lb fresh spinach

1 tsp onion powder

1 cup mozzarella cheese, shredded

7.5 oz cream cheese, cubed

1/2 cup mayonnaise

1/2 cup sour cream

1/2 cup chicken broth

1 tbsp olive oil

2 garlic cloves, minced

1/4 tsp pepper

1/2 tsp salt

Directions:

Add oil into the Pressure Pot and set the pot on sauté mode.

Add spinach and garlic and sauté until spinach is wilted. Drain excess liquid.

Add remaining ingredients and stir well.

Seal pot with lid and cook on manual high pressure for 4 minutes.

Once done then release pressure using the quick-release method then open the lid.

Stir well and serve.

Nutrition:

Calories 179, Fat 15.9g, Carbohydrates 6.1g, Sugar 1.1g, Protein 4.5g, Cholesterol 33mg.

Cauliflower with Greek-Style Sauce

Preparation time:10 minutes | Cooking Time: 4 minutes

Servings 4

Ingredients:

1 ½ pounds cauliflower, broken into florets

1/2 cup vegetable stock, preferably homemade

1 tablespoon peanut oil

1 tablespoon fresh parsley, chopped

1/2 cup Greek-style yogurt

1 teaspoon curry powder

1 habanero pepper, minced

1 yellow onion, chopped

1 clove garlic, pressed

1 tablespoon fresh cilantro, chopped

Sea salt, to taste

2 tomatoes, puréed

1/2 teaspoon ground black pepper

1/2 teaspoon red pepper flakes

Directions:

Press the "Sauté" button to heat your Pressure Pot. Now, heat the oil and sauté the onion for 1 to 2 minutes.

Add the garlic and continue to cook until fragrant.

Stir in the remaining ingredients, except the yogurt; stir to combine well.

Secure the lid. Choose the "Manual" mode and High pressure; cook for 3 minutes. Once cooking is complete, use a quick pressure release; carefully remove the lid.

Pour in the yogurt, stir well, and serve immediately.

Nutrition:

Calories 121, Fat 6.6g, Carbs 13.4g, Protein 4.8g, Sugars 5.8g.

Salted Peanuts

Preparation Time: 10 minutes | Cooking Time: 10 minutes | Servings: 4

Ingredients:

1 cup peanuts

2 tbsp olive oil

Salt

Directions:

In a bowl, toss peanuts, oil, and salt.

Place the dehydrating tray in a multi-level air fryer basket and place basket in the Pressure Pot.

Spread peanuts on a dehydrating tray.

Seal pot with air fryer lid and select air fry mode then set the temperature to 320° F and timer for 10 minutes. Stir halfway through.

Serve and enjoy.

Nutrition:

Calories 267, Fat 25g, Carbohydrates 5.9g, Sugar 1.5g, Protein 9.4g, Cholesterol 0mg.

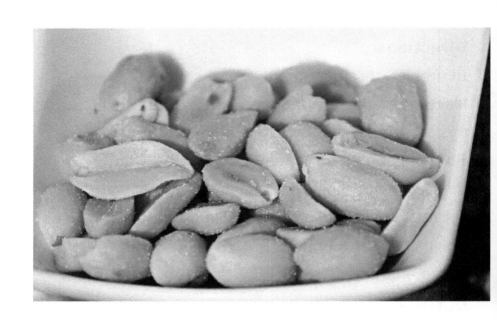

Potato Wedges

Preparation Time: 10 minutes | Cooking Time: 24 minutes | Servings: 2

Ingredients:

1/2 lb potatoes, cut into wedges

1 tbsp olive oil

Pepper

Salt

Directions:

In a bowl, toss potato wedges with oil, pepper, and salt. Spray Pressure Pot multi-level air fryer basket with cooking spray.

Potato wedges into the air fryer basket and place basket into the Pressure Pot.

Seal pot with air fryer lid and select air fry mode then set the temperature to 390° F and timer for 24 minutes. Stir halfway through.

Serve and enjoy.

Nutrition:

Calories 138, Fat 7.1g, Carbs 17.9g, Sugar 1.3g, Protein 1.9g, Cholesterol 0mg.

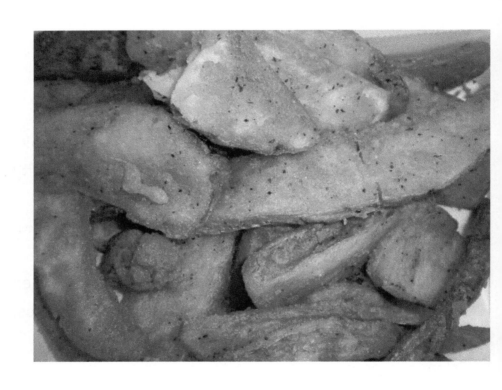

Ranch Chickpeas

Preparation Time: 10 minutes | Cooking Time: 12 minutes | Servings: 4

Ingredients:

14 oz can chickpeas, rinsed, drained and pat dry

1 1/2 tsp ranch seasoning mix

Pepper

Salt

Directions:

Add chickpeas, ranch seasoning, pepper, and salt into the mixing bowl and toss well.

Place the dehydrating tray in a multi-level air fryer basket and place basket in the Pressure Pot.

Spread chickpeas on a dehydrating tray.

Seal pot with air fryer lid and select air fry mode then set the temperature to 375° F and timer for 12 minutes.

Stir halfway through.

Serve and enjoy.

Nutrition:

Calories 120, Fat 1.1g, Carbohydrates 22.5g, Sugar 0g, Protein 4.9g, Cholesterol 0mg.

Radish Chips

Preparation Time: 10 minutes | Cooking Time: 12 minutes | Servings: 2

Ingredients:

1/2 lb radishes, sliced thinly

1/2 tsp red pepper flakes, crushed

1/2 tbsp olive oil

1/2 tbsp lime juice

Pepper

Salt

Directions:

Add radish slices and remaining ingredients into the mixing bowl and toss well.

Spray Pressure Pot multi-level air fryer basket with cooking spray.

Add radish slices into the air fryer basket and place basket into the Pressure Pot.

Seal pot with air fryer lid and select air fry mode then set the temperature to 380° F and timer for 12 minutes.

Stir halfway through.

Serve and enjoy.

Nutrition:

Calories 52, Fat 3.7g, Carbohydrates 5.1g, Sugar 2.4g, Protein 0.9g, Cholesterol 0mg.

Cream Cheese Brownies

Preparation time: 35 minutes | Cooking Time: 40 minutes | Servings: 6

Ingredients:

3 eggs, whisked

¼ cup almond flour

¼ cup coconut flour

½ cup almond milk

2 tbsp. Cocoa powder

3 tbsp. Swerve

6 tbsp. Cream cheese, soft

3 tbsp. Coconut oil; melted

1 tsp. Vanilla extract

¼ tsp. Baking soda

Cooking spray

Directions:

Grease a cake pan that fits the air fryer with the cooking spray.

Take a bowl and mix rest of the ingredients, whisk well and pour into the pan

Put the pan in your air fryer, cook at 370°f for 25 minutes, cool the brownies down, slice, and serve.

Nutrition:

Calories 182, Fat 12g, Fiber 2g, Carbs 4g, Protein 6g.

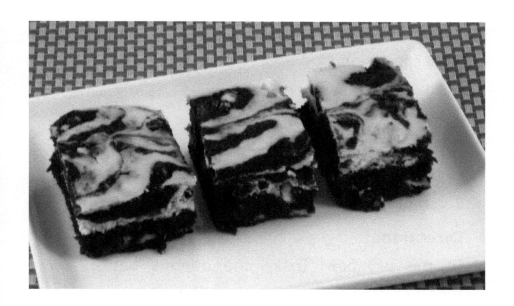

Cinnamon Muffins

Preparation Time: 10 minutes | Cooking Time: 18 minutes | Servings: 4

Ingredients:

4 teaspoons cream cheese

1 teaspoon ground cinnamon

1 tablespoon butter, softened

1 egg, beaten

4 teaspoons almond flour

½ teaspoon baking powder

1 teaspoon lemon juice

2 scoops stevia

¼ teaspoon vanilla extract

1 cup of water, for cooking

Directions:

In the big bowl make the muffins batter: mix up together cream cheese, ground cinnamon, butter, egg, almond flour, baking powder, lemon juice, stevia, and vanilla extract.

When the mixture is smooth and thick, pour it into the 4 muffin molds.

Then pour the water into the Pressure Pot and insert the trivet.

Place the muffins on the trivet and close the lid.

Cook them for 18 minutes on Manual mode (high pressure).

When the time is over, make a quick pressure release and cool the cooked muffins well.

Nutrition:

Calories 216, fat 19.2g, fiber 3.3g, carbs 7g, protein 7.7g.

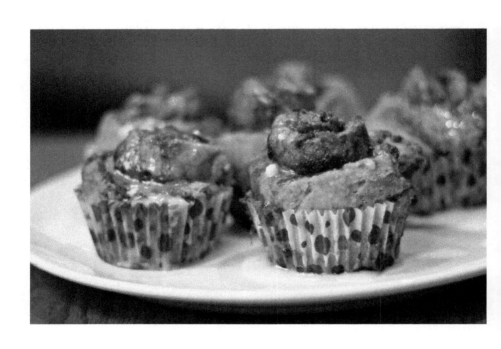

Keto Fudge

Preparation Time: 10 minutes | Cooking Time: 6 minutes | Servings: 5

Ingredients:

¾ cup of cocoa powder

1 oz dark chocolate

4 tablespoons butter

1 tablespoon ricotta cheese

¼ teaspoon vanilla extract

Directions:

Preheat the Pressure Pot on sauté mode for 3 minutes.

Place chocolate in the Pressure Pot.

Add butter and ricotta cheese.

Then add vanilla extract and cook the ingredients until you get a liquid mixture.

Then add cocoa powder and whisk it to avoid the lumps.

Line the glass mold with baking paper and pour the hot liquid mixture inside.

Flatten it gently.

Refrigerate it until solid.

Then cut/crack the cooked fudge into the serving pieces.

Nutrition:

Calories 155, fat 13.8g, fiber 4.6g, carbs 10.7g, protein 3.3g.

Fluffy Donuts

Preparation Time: 20 minutes | Cooking Time: 14 minutes | Servings: 2

Ingredients:

1 tablespoon organic almond milk

1 egg, beaten

¼ teaspoon baking powder

¼ teaspoon apple cider vinegar

1 teaspoon ghee, melted

1 teaspoon vanilla extract

1 tablespoon Erythritol

¾ teaspoon xanthan gum

1 teaspoon flax meal

1 scoop stevia

¼ teaspoon ground nutmeg

1 tablespoon almond flour

1 cup water, for cooking

Directions:

Make the dough for the donut: in the big bowl mix up almond milk, egg, baking powder, apple cider vinegar, ghee, vanilla extract, Erythritol, xanthan gum, flax meal, and almond flour.

With the help of the spoon stir the mixture gently. Then knead the non-sticky dough.

Cut it into small pieces and put it in the silicone donut molds.

Pour water and insert the trivet in the Pressure Pot.

Place the silicone molds with donuts on the trivet and close the lid.

Cook the donuts on manual mode "high pressure" for 14 minutes.

When the time is over, make a quick pressure release and open the lid.

In the shallow bowl mix up together ground nutmeg and stevia.

Sprinkle every donut with the stevia mixture.

Nutrition:

Calories 233, fat 18.9g, fiber 5.4g, carbs 9.3g, protein 9.1g.

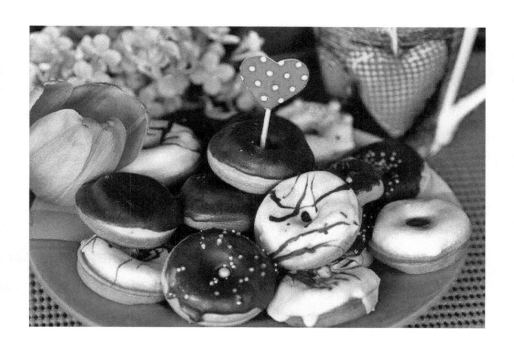

Coconut Muffins

Preparation Time: 15 minutes | Cooking Time: 12 minutes | Servings: 6

Ingredients:

½ cup coconut flour

2 eggs, beaten

¼ cup Splenda

½ teaspoon vanilla extract

3 teaspoons coconut flakes

¼ cup heavy cream

1 teaspoon baking powder

1 teaspoon lemon zest, grated

1 cup water, for cooking

Directions:

Make the muffin batter: In the bowl whisk together coconut flour, eggs, Splenda, vanilla extract, coconut flour, heavy cream, baking powder, and lemon zest.

Use the hand blender to make the batter smooth.

Then pour water into the Pressure Pot and insert the trivet.

Pour muffins batter in the muffin molds.

Then transfer the molds on the trivet and close the lid.

Cook the desert on manual mode (high pressure for 12 minutes.

When the time is over, allow the natural pressure release for 5 minutes.

Nutrition:

Calories 48, fat 3.8g, fiber 0.7g, carbs 1.9g, protein 2.2g.

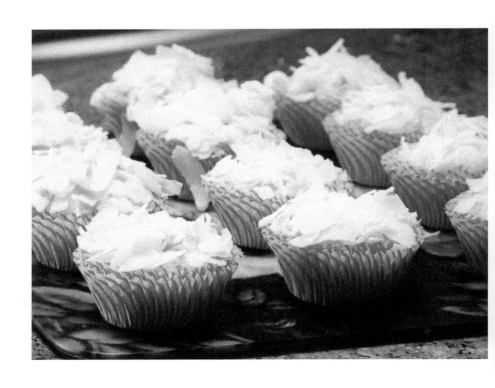

Raspberry Pie

Preparation Time: 15 minutes | Cooking Time: 25 minutes | Servings: 6

Ingredients:

¼ cup raspberries

1 tablespoon Erythritol

3 tablespoons butter, softened

¼ teaspoon baking powder

½ cup almond flour

1 tablespoon flax meal

1 teaspoon ghee, melted

1 cup water, for cooking

Directions:

Blend raspberries with Erythritol in the blender until smooth.

Then in the mixing bowl combine butter, baking powder, almond flour, flax meal, and knead the dough.

Cut it into 2 pieces.

Then put one piece of dough in the freezer.

Meanwhile, roll up the remaining piece of dough in the shape of a circle.

Grease the Pressure Pot baking mold with ghee.

Place the dough circle in the prepared baking mold.

Then pour the blended raspberry mixture over it.

Flatten it with the help of the spoon.

Then grate the frozen piece of dough over the raspberries.

Pour water and insert the trivet in the Pressure Pot.

Cover the pie with foil and put it on the trivet.

Close the lid and cook the pie on manual mode (high pressure for 25 minutes.

When the time is finished, make a quick pressure release.

Discard the foil from the pie and let it cool to room temperature.

Nutrition:

Calories 118, fat 11.6g, fiber 1.7g, carbs 3g, protein 2.4g.

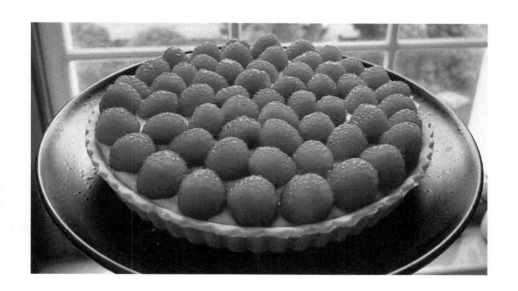

Mint Cookies

Preparation Time: 10 minutes | Cooking Time: 15 minutes | Servings: 4

Ingredients:

¼ cup Erythritol

½ teaspoon dried mint

¼ teaspoon mint extract

4 teaspoons cocoa powder

2 egg whites

¼ teaspoon baking powder

¼ teaspoon lemon juice

1 cup water, for cooking

Directions:

Whisk the egg whites gently and add dried mint.

Then add Erythritol, mint extract, cocoa powder, baking powder, and lemon juice.

Stir the mass until smooth.

Pour water into the Pressure Pot.

Line the Pressure Pot trivet with the baking paper.

Place it in the Pressure Pot.

With the help of the scooper make 4 cookies and put them on the trivet.

Close the lid and cook the cookies on manual mode (high pressure for 15 minutes.

When the time is over, make a quick pressure release.

Open the lid and transfer the cookies to the plate or chopping board.

Cool the cookies well.

Nutrition:

Calories 13, fat 0.3g, fiber 0.6g, carbs 1.3g, protein 2.1g.

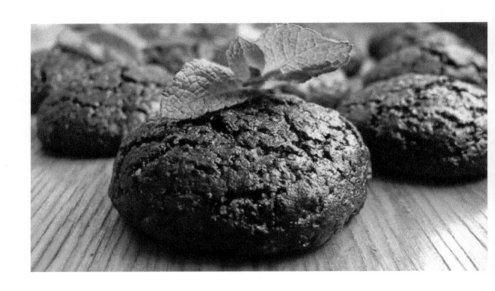

Coconut Clouds

Preparation Time: 10 minutes | Cooking Time: 6 minutes | Servings:2

Ingredients:

2 egg whites

4 tablespoons coconut flakes

1 tablespoon almond meal

¼ teaspoon ghee

1 teaspoon Erythritol

Directions:

Whisk the egg whites until strong peaks.

Then slowly add the almond meal and coconut flakes.

Add Erythritol and stir the mixture until homogenous with the help of the silicone spatula.

Toss ghee in the Pressure Pot and preheat it on sauté mode for 2 minutes.

Then with the help of the spoon, make the clouds from the egg white mixture and put them in the hot ghee.

Close the lid and cook the dessert on sauté mode for 4 minutes.

Nutrition:

Calories 74, fat 5.4g, fiber 1.3g, carbs 2.4g, protein 4.6g.

Shortbread Cookies

Preparation Time: 15 minutes | Cooking Time: 14 minutes | Servings: 6

Ingredients:

1 egg, beaten

¾ teaspoon salt

1 tablespoon almond butter

1 teaspoon coconut oil

¼ teaspoon baking powder

¼ teaspoon apple cider vinegar

1 tablespoon Erythritol

5 oz coconut flour

1 cup water, for cooking

Directions:

Mix up egg with salt, almond butter, coconut flour, and baking powder.

Add apple cider vinegar, coconut oil, and Erythritol.

Knead the dough and make 6 balls from it.

Then press the balls gently with the help of the hand palm and place in the non-sticky Pressure Pot baking tray.

Pour water and insert the trivet in the Pressure Pot.

Place the tray with cookies on the trivet and close the lid.

Cook the cookies on manual mode (high pressure for 14 minutes.

When the time is over, make a quick pressure release and open the lid.

Transfer the cooked cookies to the plate and let them cool well.

Nutrition:

Calories 135, fat 5.5g, fiber 10.4g, carbs 17.5g, protein 4.9g.

Lime Bars

Preparation Time: 20 minutes | Cooking Time: 10 minutes | Servings: 6

Ingredients:

½ cup coconut flour

2 teaspoons coconut oil

¼ teaspoon baking powder

½ tablespoon cream cheese

1/3 cup coconut cream

2 tablespoons lime juice

1 teaspoon lime zest, grated

2 tablespoons Erythritol

1 cup water, for cooking

Directions:

Knead the dough from coconut flour, coconut oil, baking powder, and cream cheese.

When the mixture is soft and non-sticky, it is prepared.

Then line the Pressure Pot bowl with baking paper.

Place the dough inside and flatten it in the shape of the pie crust (make the edges).

Close the lid and cook it on sauté mode for 5 minutes.

After this, switch off the Pressure Pot.

Make the filling: mix up coconut cream, lime juice, lime zest, and Erythritol.

Then pour the liquid over the cooked pie crust and cook it in sauté mode for 5 minutes more.

When the time is over, transfer the cooked meal to the freezer for 10 minutes.

Cut the dessert into bars.

Nutrition:

Calories 88, fat 6g, fiber 4.3g, carbs 7.9g, protein 1.7g.

Peppermint Cookies

Preparation Time: 20 minutes | Cooking Time: 5 minutes | Servings: 2

Ingredients:

¼ teaspoon peppermint extract

2 tablespoons almond flour

1 teaspoon heavy cream

½ teaspoon butter softened

¼ oz dark chocolate

Directions:

Preheat the Pressure Pot on sauté mode for 3 minutes.

Then add almond flour, butter, and heavy cream.

Add peppermint extract and dark chocolate.

Sauté the mixture for 2 minutes. Stir well.

Then line the tray with baking paper.

With the help of the spoon make the cookies from the peppermint mixture and transfer them to the prepared baking paper.

Refrigerate the cookies for 20 minutes.

Nutrition:

Calories 199, fat 17.1g, fiber 3.3g, carbs 8.1g, protein 6.2g.

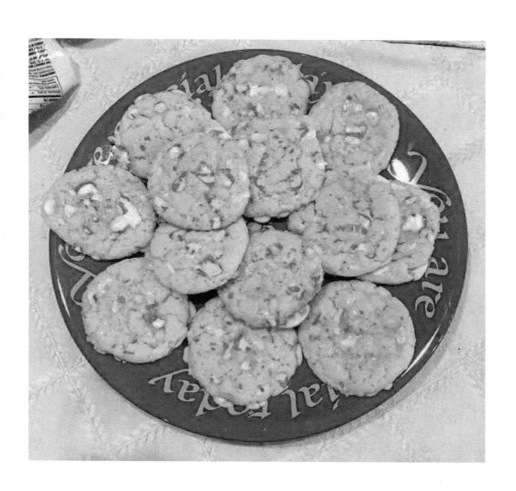

Toffee Cookie

Preparation Time: 10 minutes | Cooking Time: 9 minutes | Servings: 12

Ingredients:

1 egg

1/3 cup toffee chips

1/2 tsp baking powder

1 cup all-purpose flour

1 tsp vanilla

1/2 cup brown sugar

4 tbsp butter, softened

1/8 tsp salt

Directions:

In a mixing bowl, beat butter and sugar until smooth.

Add egg and vanilla and stir to combine.

Add flour, baking powder, and salt and stir to combine.

Add toffee chips and stir to combine. Place cookie mixture into the refrigerator for 1 hour.

Place the dehydrating tray in a multi-level air fryer basket and place basket in the Pressure Pot.

Line dehydrating tray with parchment paper.

Make cookies from the mixture and place some cookies on the dehydrating tray.

Seal pot with air fryer lid and select bake mode then set the temperature to 350° F and timer for 9 minutes.

Bake remaining cookies using the same method.

Serve and enjoy.

Nutrition:

Calories 107, Fat 4.6g, Carbohydrates 14.6g, Sugar 6.5g, Protein 1.7g, Cholesterol 24mg.

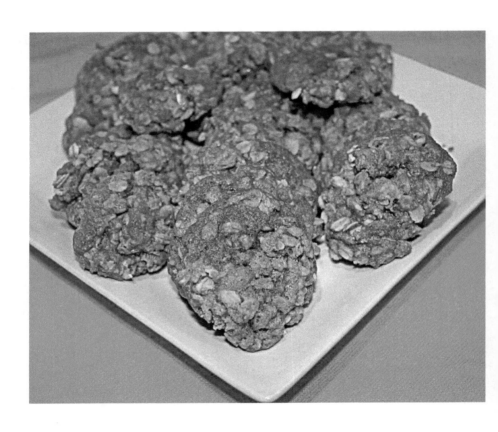

Vanilla Strawberry Cobbler

Preparation Time: 10 minutes | Cooking Time: 12 minutes | Servings: 2

Ingredients:

1/2 cup strawberries, sliced

1 1/4 cup all-purpose flour

3/4 cup milk

1 1/2 tsp baking powder

1/2 cup sugar

1/2 tsp vanilla

1/3 cup butter

Directions:

In a mixing bowl, add all ingredients except strawberries and mix well.

Add strawberries and fold well.

Spray 3 ramekins with cooking spray then pour batter into the ramekins.

Pour 1 1/2 cups water into the inner pot of Pressure Pot duo crisp then place steamer rack into the pot.

Place ramekins on top of the steamer rack.

Seal the pot with a pressure-cooking lid and cook on high for 12 minutes.

Once done, allow to release pressure naturally. Remove lid.

Serve and enjoy.

Nutrition:

Calories 807, Fat 33.5g, Carbohydrates 118.8g, Sugar 56.2g, Protein 11.6g, Cholesterol 89mg.

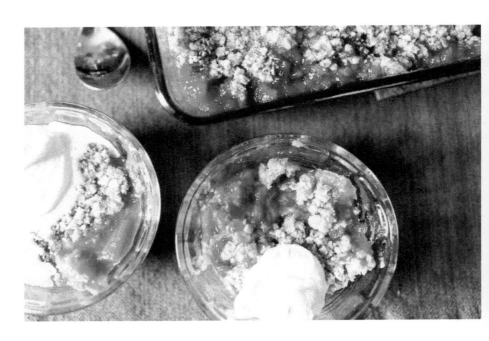

Cinnamon Peach Cobbler

Preparation Time: 10 minutes | Cooking Time: 10 minutes | Servings: 6

Ingredients:

20 oz can peach pie filling

1 1/2 tsp cinnamon

1/2 cup butter, melted

15 oz vanilla cake mix

1 tsp nutmeg

Directions:

Spray inner pot of Pressure Pot duo crisp with cooking spray.

Add peach pie filling into the pot.

In a mixing bowl, mix the remaining ingredients and sprinkle over peaches.

Seal the pot with a pressure-cooking lid and cook on high for 10 minutes.

Once done, release pressure using a quick release. Remove lid.

Serve and enjoy.

Nutrition:

Calories 453, Fat 15.5g, Carbohydrates 78g, Sugar 48.7g, Protein 0.2g, Cholesterol 41mg.

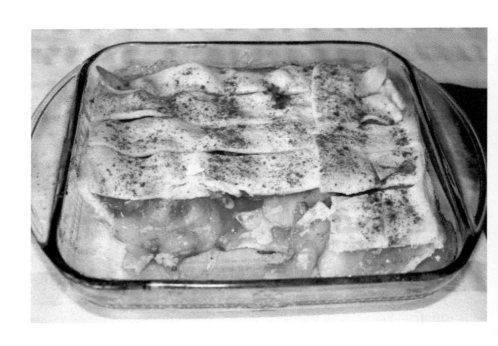

Pear Apple Crisp

Preparation Time: 10 minutes | Cooking Time: 10 minutes | Servings: 4

Ingredients:

2 pears, cut into chunks

4 apples, peel, and cut into chunks

3/4 tsp cinnamon

1/4 cup date syrup

1 cup steel-cut oats

1 1/2 cup hot water

Directions:

Add all ingredients into the inner pot of Pressure Pot duo crisp and stir well.

Seal the pot with a pressure-cooking lid and cook on high for 10 minutes.

Once done, allow to release pressure naturally.

Remove lid.

Serve and enjoy.

Nutrition:

Calories 273, Fat 1.9g, Carbohydrates 65.4g, Sugar 37.7g, Protein 3.8g, Cholesterol 0mg.

Cherry Black Rice Pudding

Preparation Time: 10 minutes | Cooking Time: 22 minutes | Servings: 3

Ingredients:

2 eggs

1 cup black rice, rinsed

3/4 cup half and half

1/2 cup sugar

1 cup milk

1 tbsp butter

2/3 cup dried cherries

1 tsp vanilla

1 1/2 cups water

1/4 tsp salt

Directions:

Add rice, butter, salt, and water into the inner pot of Pressure Pot duo crisp and stir well.

Seal the pot with a pressure-cooking lid and cook on high for 22 minutes.

Once done, allow to release pressure naturally. Remove lid.

Add milk and sugar and stir well.

Set Pressure Pot on sauté, mode cook, until sugar is dissolved.

Whisk eggs with vanilla and half and a half and pour through a strainer into the pot.

Stir constantly until begins to boil. Turn off the pot.

Add cherries and stir well and serve.

Nutrition:

Calories 406, Fat 15.7g, Carbohydrates 57.9g, Sugar 37.8g, Protein 10.6g, Cholesterol 149mg.

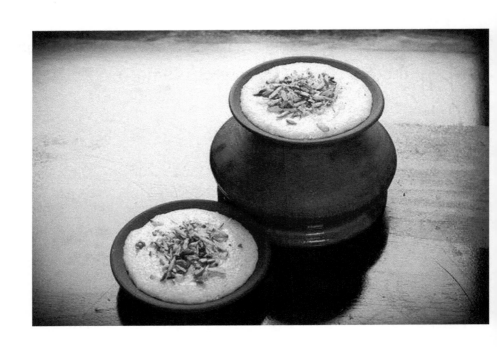

Apple Pie Pudding

Preparation Time: 10 minutes | Cooking Time: 5 minutes | Servings: 4

Ingredients:

4 cups of rice

1/4 cup raisins

1 tbsp apple pie spice

2 cup almond milk

3 1/2 cups apples, chopped

1/4 tsp cardamom

1 tbsp vanilla

Directions:

Add all ingredients into the inner pot of Pressure Pot duo crisp and stir well.

Seal the pot with a pressure-cooking lid and cook on high for 5 minutes.

Once done, release pressure using a quick release. Remove lid.

Stir well and serve.

Nutrition:

Calories 1094, Fat 30.4g, Carbohydrates 190.2g, Sugar 30.4g, Protein 16.8g, Cholesterol 0mg.

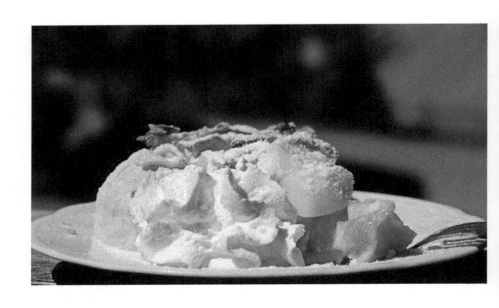

French Toast Bites

Preparation time: 5 minutes | Cooking Time: 15 minutes | Servings: 8

Ingredients:

Almond milk

Cinnamon

Sweetener

3 eggs

4 pieces of wheat bread

Directions:

Preparing the ingredients. Preheat the instant crisp air fryer to 360° F.

Whisk eggs and thin out with almond milk.

Mix 1/3 cup of sweetener with lots of cinnamon.

Tear bread in half, ball up pieces, and press together to form a ball.

Soak bread balls in egg and then roll into cinnamon sugar, making sure to thoroughly coat.

Air frying. Place coated bread balls into the instant crisp air fryer, close the air fryer lid.

Select bake and bake for 15 minutes.

Nutrition:

Calories 289, Fat 11g, Protein 0g, Sugar 4g.

Lightning Source UK Ltd.
Milton Keynes UK
UKHW021014240621
386072UK00001B/56